The Caregiver's Guide
To Less Stress!

A Quick & Easy Way to Reduce Your Daily Stress

by

Carol L Rickard, LCSW

America's Ultimate Stress Expert

As Featured:

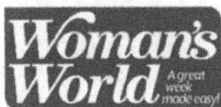

Reader's digest

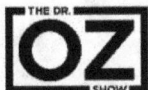

DR.OZ
THE GOOD LIFE

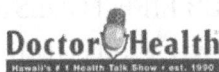

The Caregiver's Guide to Less Stress
by Carol L Rickard, LCSW

© 2019 Carol L Rickard   All Rights Reserved

All rights reserved. No part of this book may be reproduced for resale, redistribution, or any other purposes (including but not limited to eBooks, pamphlets, articles, video or audiotapes, & handouts or slides for lectures or workshops). Permission to reproduce these materials for those and any other purposes must be obtained in writing from the author.

The author & publisher of this book do not dispense medical advice nor prescribe the use of this material as a form of treatment. The author & publisher are not engaged in rendering psychological, medical, or other professional services. The purpose of this material is educational only.

ISBN: 978-1-947745-18-6   (paperback)
ISBN: 978-1-947745-19-3   (Ebook)

Published by:

Well YOUniversity Publications
A Division of Well YOUniversity, LLC
5 Zion Rd.
Hopewell, NJ 08525
888 LIFE TOOLS (543-3866)
www.WellYOUniversity.com

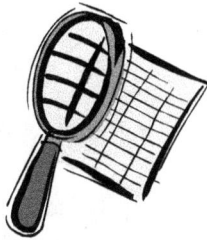

What will you get out of this book?

- A better understanding of WHY you must take action to reduce & manage your daily stress as a caregiver.

- A simple & practical system that will decrease your STRESS levels in just 60 seconds or less!

- Improved health & wellbeing because you know how to **keep STRESS from ruining it!**

Table of Contents

Sign Up For…

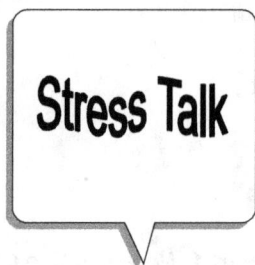

This 5-minute video newsletter will give you

more tips, tools, & rules for taking control of…

STRESS!

Sign up at:

StressYOUniversity.com/Stress-Talk

Welcome

Caregivers are the most at risk

group when it comes to …

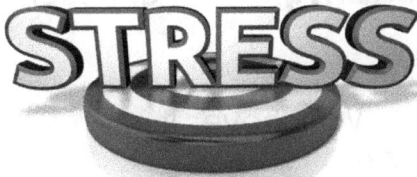

Even when you *CHOOSE* to be one!

It can be **fulfilling & special role**

And yet

one of the **MOST** *stressful* as well.

If you are reading this , there is

one thing I know for sure about you…

You are either...

at a breaking point

OR

heading in that direction.

Whichever it is –

I am glad you are here!

There is NO *shortage* when it comes

to caregiver stress!

From navigating doctors & dealing with

insurance to having to DO IT ALL

while still working to just everyday life...

There's plenty to go around & be shared.

2

The problem…

When **stress** is not managed,

it has the *power to ruin* a lot of things…

health

relationships

hopes

dreams

&… careers.

It is my sincere hope you will take &

use what you learn in this book!

You will either manage your stress

or

IT CONTINUES TO MANAGE YOU!

Getting Started

Let me ask you a **?** ■■■

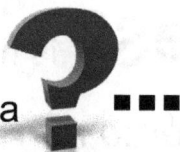

What if you could learn how to

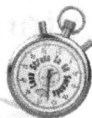

eliminate stress in just *60 seconds*?

Would you want to know?

If the answer is **"yes"**

than just keep on reading!

You are about to learn a **revolutionary**

approach to managing your stress.

4

This approach will put **you** in

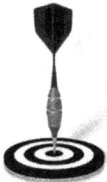

control of stress once & for all.

It may seem like it is too good to be true –

But *it isn't!*

I'm going to share with you the

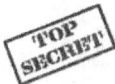

secret system I've been

teaching my patients since 1991.

Equally as important,

it is the **same system** I use every day...

I LIVE WHAT I TEACH!

That wasn't always the case…

When I started 17 years ago at the

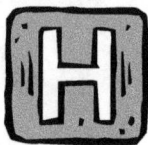

where I still currently work –

STRESS had *control* of me!

Only…

I didn't *realize* it...

It wasn't until I landed

in my doctor's office

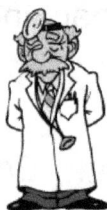

3 weeks in a row

with *horrible migraines* & he asked

"Carol, what's got you so stressed?"

Now, the most **embarrassing** part:

Here I was *teaching my patients*

the

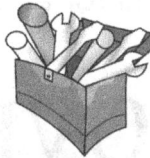

to manage their stress…

BUT I wasn't *using them myself!*

Since that day,

I have **kept** my commitment to

I LIVE WHAT I TEACH every day!

Everything I share here with you –

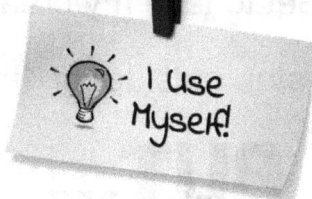

 I use Myself!

My Biggest Excuse

I'd been in my new job at the

hospital for about 8 months.

I LOVED IT!

In fact, I remember thinking to myself:

*'I can't believe I am
getting paid to do this!'*

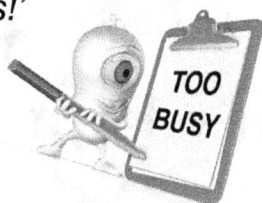

TOO
BUSY

It was a busy place – so busy I didn't…

Get to stop & eat lunch

Get to take my breaks

Even step outside for 1 minute!

BUT...

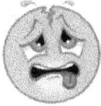

When the migraines hit me so HARD I knew I had to make a

Big change.

Leaving my job was not an option.

Besides –

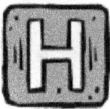

I knew from having worked at other hospitals, it would be the same *STRESS everywhere.*

What had to **change was ME!**
I had to start using the tools I was teaching even if I only had *60* seconds.

That's how I *discovered my system works!*

About This Book

I doubt you have read a [book] like this!

I like to use a lot of pictures, analogies, & word art which help information stick in the brain!

I call my approach:

SMARTheory™

(It's what makes my books and services *different* from all others!)

There are two parts to this book:

Part 1: Now You See It! ☺☺

Part 2: Now You Don't!

Part 1: Now You See It!

Here I introduce you to a concept

that will **CHANGE**

your life **forever**....

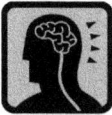

You'll never think about stress

the same way **again!**

You also learn WHY *we must*

DO something about stress.

Did you know...

Studies show over 80% of people

DO NOTHING about

their record high stress levels.

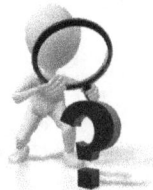

Part Two: Now You Don't

This section will *give* YOU the

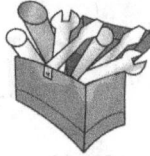

You'll learn **A LOT** of

different "tools"!

The secret I learned a long time ago…

Having the *right tool*

for the *right job* makes

the difference between

success and failure.

Also, **1** TOOL won't work
the same for everyone!

What's The Impact?

Stress can be found *all around the world.*

Caregivers are at **epidemic** levels -

just look at some of the headlines:

Caregiving Stress --
Hazardous to Your Health
and Sometimes Deadly
December 11, 2007

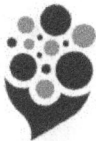

CANADIAN
PUBLIC HEALTH
ASSOCIATION

JANUARY 26, 2016

Caregiver burden takes
a toll on mental health

TODAY'S
CAREGIVER

February 21, 2018 10:31 AM

**Cost, Uncertainty and Stress Plague
Long-Distance Caregivers**
by Maureen Hewitt

US Population Statistics: (APA / AIS 7/28/14)

77%
Regularly experience physical
symptoms caused by stress

54%
Say stress has caused them to
fight with those they love.

76%
Identify money and work as
the leading cause of stress

48%
Say stress has had a negative
impact on their lives

$300 Billion
Estimated annual cost to US
businesses / employers

So, what does this mean?

Stress is a... **HUGE** problem

The **?** is:

What is stress COSTING YOU?

Are you so stressed out you can't sleep?

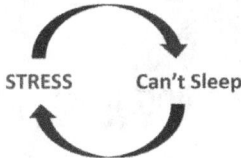

STRESS   Can't Sleep

Is your stress spilling out on the wrong
people or following you to work?

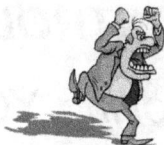

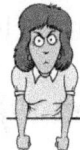

Is stress affecting your work?

Are you starting to have health issues?

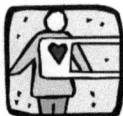

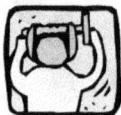

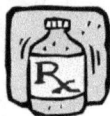

A "yes" to any of these is a sure sign
stress has taken *CONTROL* of your life

There's **good** news!

You're reading this

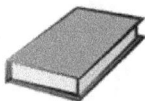

By the time you are finished…

You'll be able to **CONTROL IT**

rather than *it controlling YOU!*

It's In The Cards!

When you come to my live seminars,

as you take your seat, you'll be handed

a playing card!

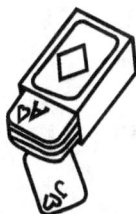

It may be a king or it may be a three….

The

key point

is:

You **DON'T** get to **CHOOSE**

what card you get!

This applies so wonderfully **to LIFE** –

where we'll face many situations that

WE DON'T GET TO CHOOSE!

This is particularly the case

when you are a caregiver.

There are **many** days where you may

have a plan for how the day will go

and **it goes the other way.**

There are so many factors

you don't get to control…..

Another person's behavior

Hospitalizations

Family members

Insurance plans

Treatment providers

So,

what are you supposed to do?

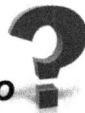

All that you *can* do…

Play the cards you're dealt that day

the **BEST** that you can!

Here's a couple of the tools I've used:

IT'S NOT

WHAT HAPPENS

TO YOU,

BUT

HOW YOU REACT

TO IT

THAT MATTERS

EPICTETUS

Another way to think about it....

We don't get to control the events,

We *do get to control*

<u>our</u> <u>response</u> to them!

We are 100% responsible for our **choice:**

Controlling

How

Our

Intentions

Create

Experiences

© 2019 & licensed by Well YOUniversity, LLC
Taken from the *WordTools Series*

This is my favorite &

the *MOST* POWERFUL:

WHEN WE FACE A SITUATION

THAT *CANNOT* BE CHANGED

WE ARE **CHALLENGED**
TO

CHANGE OURSELVES

VICTOR FRANKL

Are you trying to change things

you CAN'T CONTROL?

Do the exercise on the next page to see!

Write down as many things you can think

of having to do with caregiving:

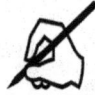

(Use another piece of paper if you need more room!)

Now go back & circle

ONLY the things **you can** control!

Tracking Your Progress

Monitoring

I developed a tool to help my patients

be able to track their progress.

The Stressometer™

It's pretty simple to use!

1st - Read each question & select the
answer that *best describes* you.

2nd - When you get to the end, *total up*
all the numbers for a score

3rd - *Check your score* on the key.
Repeat to see how you progress!

24

The Stressometer

I find when I try to go to sleep, my mind just keeps racing about things.

1	2	3	4	5	6	7

Not at all   All the time

I find my appetite changes, I'm either eating more or eating less.

1	2	3	4	5	6	7

Not at all   All the time

I find myself getting really angry over the littlest things.

1	2	3	4	5	6	7

Not at all   All the time

I find I am having increased health issues. (ie. migraines, pain, & digestive)

1	2	3	4	5	6	7

Not at all   All the time

I find my relationship is being impacted by what goes on at work / home.

1	2	3	4	5	6	7

Not at all   All the time

Total: _____

How Stressed Are You?

5–10 **Great news!**

You have no stress!

11–15 **Good news!**

You have just a little bit of stress!

16–20 **Not bad!**

You seem to still have a handle on it!

21–25 **WATCH OUT!**

STRESS is *starting to cause trouble!*

26–30 **WARNING…**

STRESS is *greatly impacting* your life.

31–35 **DANGER Zone!**

Your level has you at extreme risk.

Your score ***will come down*** when
you use the system!!!

Another Tracking Tool

How to tell if this 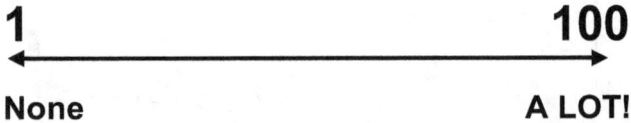 is helping!

There are 2 more ways to track -

Both use a score of 1 to 100

1   **100**

$\longleftrightarrow$

None   **A LOT!**

#1   Track your **daily** stress level
(do this every evening)

#2   Track your level **before & after** you use the tools!

**Since this is new for you
it may take a little time for you to
get used to the tools!**

In order for this system to WORK…

YOU must *take* **ACTION!**

Here are a couple of my **WordTools** to help:

$$\textbf{A}$$

$$\textbf{C}\text{ritical}$$

$$\textbf{T}\text{ask}$$

$$\textbf{I}\text{mplemented}$$

$$\textbf{O}\text{nly}$$

$$\textbf{N}\text{ow!}$$

© 2019 & licensed by Well YOUniversity, LLC

Taken from the *WordTools Series*

No "tool" will work…

if you don't **pick it up**

&

DO something with it!!

Here's my WordTool:

Direct

Opportunity

© 2019 & licensed by Well YOUniversity, LLC
Taken from the *WordTools Series*

Lastly,

When we **_DON'T_** use the "tools"

This is what happens!

D enied

O pportunity

N ot

' T rying

© 2019 & licensed by Well YOUniversity, LLC
Taken from the *WordTools Series*

Part One
Now You See It!

(Two ways to 'see' it!)

#1

Imagine this …

I hand you a big bottle of root beer

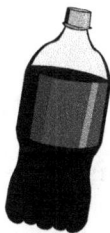

and ask you to *shake it up –*

A LOT!

Maybe you even **drop** it on the floor…

So,

what do you think will **happen**

to the bottle of root beer?

You're **right!**

The PRESSURE builds up inside!

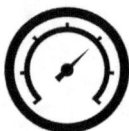

And once *the pressure gets built up*

It stays there...

It won't go away on its own.

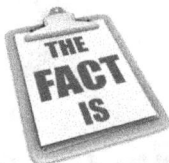

The PRESSURE doesn't go *anywhere*

UNTIL

we *do something to let it out!*

And, it's *not good* to have **too much**

PRESSURE build up inside the bottle.

Two things can happen…

#1   It comes SPILLING OUT & leaves a big mess.

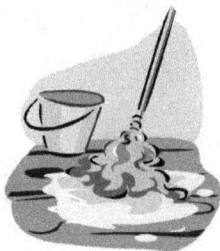

#2   It STAYS IN and ends up *ruining* the root beer.

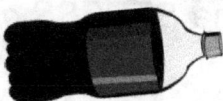

It's best to avoid both!

People are like the bottle ...

Things happen in life that

shake a person up

And…

Just like the pressure

BUILT UP

in the bottle…

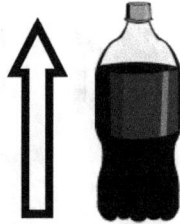

STRESS builds up *inside people!*

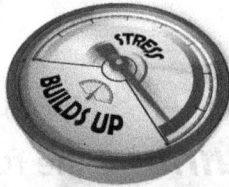

And once the *STRESS gets built up*

It stays there…

It won't go away on its own.

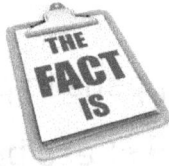

The **STRESS** doesn't go anywhere

UNTIL

we *do something to let it out!*

(we'll talk about this in part 2)

And just like the bottle,

It's *not good* for **too much**

STRESS to

build up inside people!

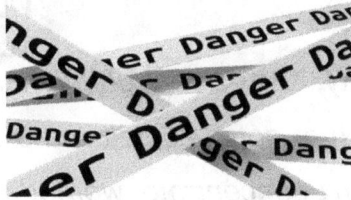

Here's what happens to people when
TOO MUCH stress builds up…

#1 It comes SPILLING OUT &
leaves a **big** mess.

Have you ever:

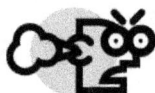

Said hurtful things or things you wished you hadn't said, yelled, got in arguments, broke things, had road rage, or slammed doors?

#2 It STAYS IN and ends up
ruining *your health.*

Have you ever:

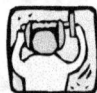

Felt anxiety, can't sleep, gotten headaches, ate too much or not at all, felt sad & depressed, couldn't concentrate, worried a lot?

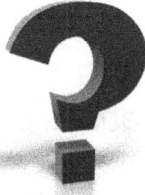

Do any of the following everyday life

things **STRESS** you out?

Chronic Pain

Bills / Finances

Looking for work

Being a caregiver

Dr's appointments

Holidays

Commute to work / school

Relationships

Not working

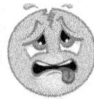

Getting sick

Family members

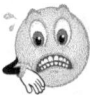
Kids / Pets

Running late or waking up lat31

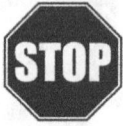

STOP **Important news:**

A situation that *causes* one person stress

may not *cause* you stress!

Now, what are the WORK things

stressing you out?

Write them down here:

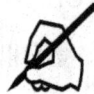

(Use another piece of paper if you need more room!)

#2

What do you think would happen if…

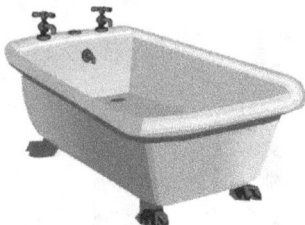

You **plugged** the drain,

turned the water **on**,

and then *walked away*?

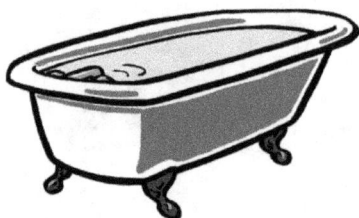

Eventually….

It would **overflow**, right?

Once it did – there'd be a

HUGE MESS!

Does this make sense?

A tub can only hold **so much!**

Two important points:

1) Once the level starts to rise – It will KEEP rising until it is **shut off.**

2) The tub ONLY has *so much room* - It can ONLY hold *so much* then it's

OVERFLOW!!!

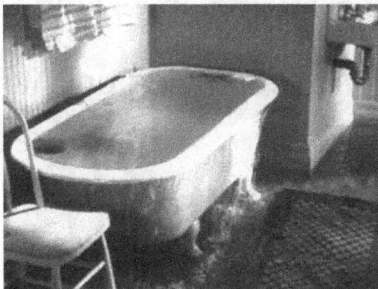

Some people think…

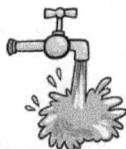

The solution is to just **turn OFF the water.**

You'll see later why this *won't* work!

When it comes to

STRESS…

People are just like a tub:

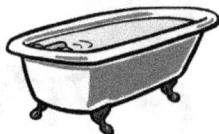

Once you wake up –

1) your **STRESS** level starts to rise

& it will keep rising until it is…

Shut off!

2) *YOU* only have *so much room* -

YOU can only hold so much

STRESS

until *YOU* will be at

OVERFLOW!!!

So,

I hope you can 👓 how

STRESS creates problems

And how it won't go away

until we…

release it!

Now that you can **SEE IT:**

Way #1

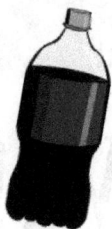

Way #2

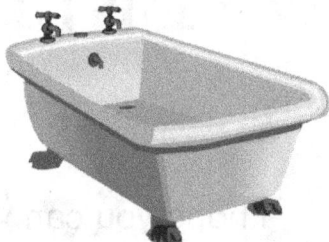

It's time to learn how to

RELEASE IT!

We're moving on to Part Two…

Part Two

Now You Don't!

(Ways to 'release' it!)

What To Do!

This is where almost everyone

gets it **wrong!**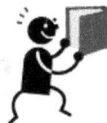

Because you're reading this book…

you'll know the

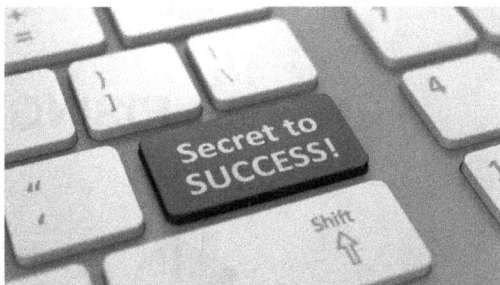

What you are about to learn is my *secret*

DO*60* System™

> ➤ It ***doesn't take*** a lot of ***time***!

> ➤ It will work for ***everyone***!

> ➤ It can be used ***everywhere***!

There are **2** steps to the

DO*60* System™

Step 1 -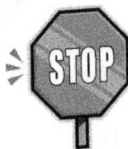

the level from **RISING!**

Step 2 -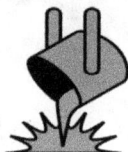

RELEASE so the level drops!

Each step must be done *in order...*

Step 1 ——→ Step 2

Each step must be done *for 60 Secs.*

Just so this makes sense…

In order to the level from **rising**

you must do something that is

calming for you!

Calming = Activities that require

NO energy or muscles

be used!

I'm afraid I have a little bit of

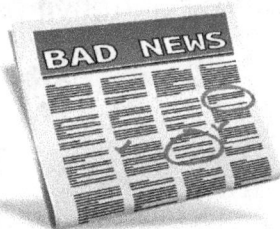

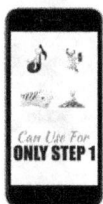

 You can *ONLY* use your cell phone

for this first step!

Cell phones **DO NOT** require

enough energy or muscles for Step Two.

Now,

In order to 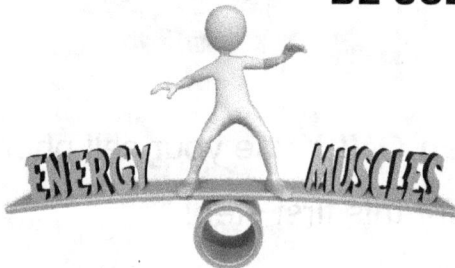 **release** & drop levels

you must do something *you like*

that is ACTIVE

Active = Activities that **DO** require

energy & muscles

BE USED!

So let's apply this

to our stress bottle…

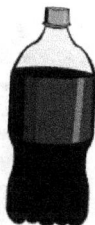

Step 1 - 🛑 **the pressure**

from continuing to build up!

Step 2 - **the pressure**

that's been built up inside!

Each step:

✓ Must be done **in order**

✓ Must be done for **60 secs.**

** Otherwise the system won't work **40

And applied to our stress tub…

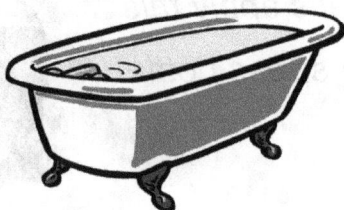

Step 1 - STOP **the level**

from continuing to rise!

Step 2 - **the level**

that's been raised already!

Where most people get it wrong…

They only *turn OFF the water.*

They **DON'T** do Step 2 - **RELEASE!**

How To Do It!
Step 1

Sign Up Today!

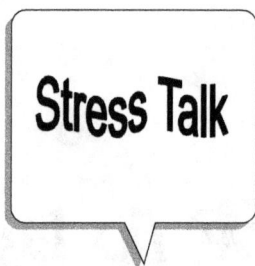

This 5 minute video newsletter will give you

more tips, tools, & rules for taking control of…

STRESS!

Sign up at:

StressYOUniversity.com/Stress-Talk

On the following pages are

a bunch of different **"tools"**.

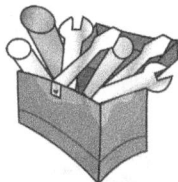

Each one is good to use for

Step 1 - STOP

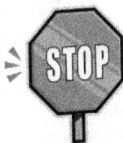

Things from **RISING!**

There are a **4 keys** to

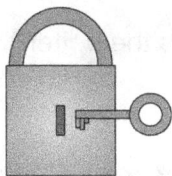

S
U
C
C
E
S
S....

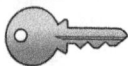

Try out each one.

(*even if* you don't think

it will work for you!)

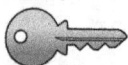

Do 60 Seconds.

(if you can go longer – *do it!*

30 secs. *is better than* none!

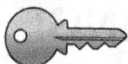

Keep a list.

(write down tools that end

up working *best for you*)

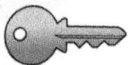

Have more than 1!

(don't set yourself up to fail

the *more tools* the better!)

You **must** do **Step 1** *before* Step 2

Step 1 ➝ Step 2

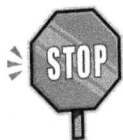 **Tool #1**

read

grab one of your favorite books

Real   **or**   **Kindle**

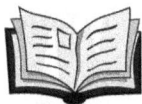   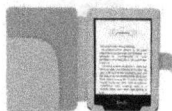

Either way….. you're reading!

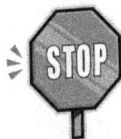 **Tool #2**

Music

Listen to one of your favorites!

Song   **or**   **Artist**

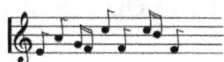   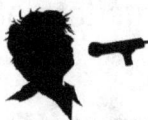

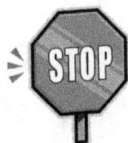

STOP **Tool #3**

Breathe

✓ **Count your breathes**

There are a couple ways to do this:

#1 **Track the # you do in 60 secs.**

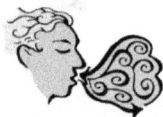

or

#2 **Set a specific # to do 10, 12, 15, 20**

Belly Breathing is best!

This gets lots of oxygen into our brain…

Oxygen is **kryptonite** to STRESS!

Another way to *BREATHE:*

✓ Square Breathing

1) **Breathe in** & count to 4 in your head (1,2,3,4)

2) **Hold it** & count to 4 in your head (1,2,3,4)

3) **Breathe out** & count to 4 in your head (1,2,3,4)

4) **Hold it** & count to 4 in your head (1,2,3,4)

5) **Repeat!**

Here's what it looks like!

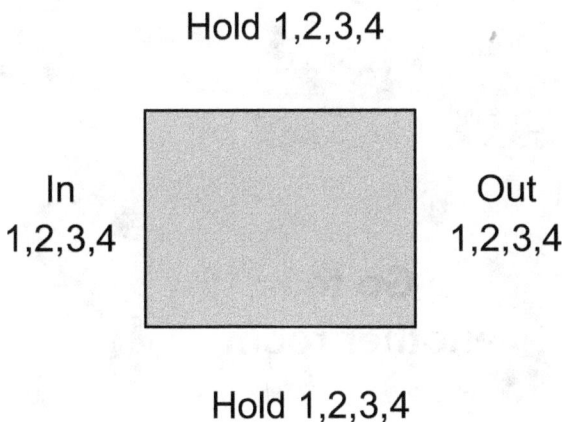

Hold 1,2,3,4

In
1,2,3,4

Out
1,2,3,4

Hold 1,2,3,4

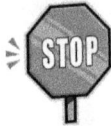 **Tool #4**

Take A Time Out

Remove yourself from the situation.

Create **space** between

YOU & the situation or person

Go outside!

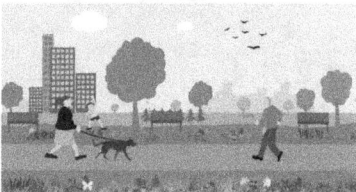

Go to another room

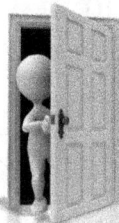

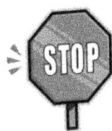

STOP **Tool #5**

Mind Push Ups!

Here's how:

1. Find a quiet spot to lie down.

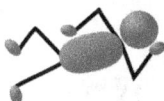

2. Set a timer for 60 secs. (*or more!*)

3. Put a book on your belly.

4. As you breathe in, make

   your belly & the book rise!

5. Breathe out like your blowing candles.

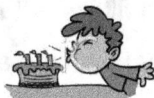

6. Repeat breathes until timer goes off!

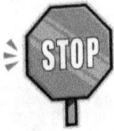

STOP **Tool #6**

+ SELF-TALK

Saying positive statements to yourself!

The 2 P's of Self-Talk!

1) Present

I AM.....
THIS IS....
I HAVE....

FUTURE

I will....
I hope...
I'm going to...

2) Positive

~~Don't~~ touch = TOUCH!

Not...
Won't...
Can't...

Our brain filters out the negative
& all we hear is what's after it: **TOUCH!**

** See a list of self-talk ideas on page 67 **

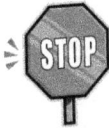

STOP Tool #7

The Serenity Prayer

God,

Grant me the **serenity** to accept
the things *I cannot change.*

The **courage** to change the things I *can.*

And the **wisdom** to know *the difference.*

Carol's
'In the Moment Serenity Prayer'

Ask yourself the following **?**

"Can I do anything about IT

RIGHT NOW?"

If yes, *DO it*!   If NO – *Let it go!*

Here's a few more *tools –*

- Guided Imagery on **YouTube**

- Count to 10 **s l o w l y !**

- Watch a favorite show or movie

- Blow bubbles

- Lie down & look at the sky

- Picture a **STOP** sign in your mind

- Make a "Calm Jar"
  Google It!

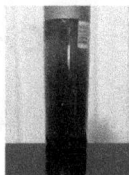

Positive Self-Talk Ideas

I no longer give power to the PAST

Today I feel peace & calm.

I am free of negative feelings.

I am learning to love myself.

Today, I choose a positive attitude.

I am terrific just the way I am!

I have all the time I need.

I am living a healthy life today

Today, I forgive all others and myself.

I am getting better one step at a time!

I am having a great day!

I am a good & caring person!

Can you think of other ways for you to:

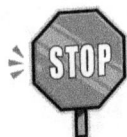

 The level from **RISING!**

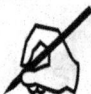

(Use another piece of paper if you need more room!)

Remember -

This step is one that is calming...

(Requires NO activity or muscles!)

How To Do It!
Step 2

Now we'll take a look at what to

do *once* you have done

Step 1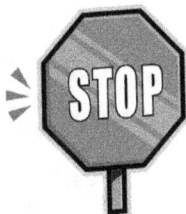

On the following pages are

more **"tools"**...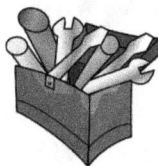

Each one of these is

good to use for

Step 2 -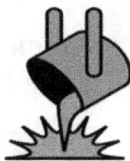

RELEASE what's there!

Again, here are those 🔑 's to success!

#1   **Try out each one.**

(**even if** you don't think

It will work for you!)

#2   **Do 60 Seconds.**

(if you can go longer – **do it!**

30 secs. **is better than** none!

#3   **Keep a list.**

(write down tools that end

up working **best for you**)

#4   **Have more than 1!**

(don't set yourself up to fail

the **more tools** the better!)

Remember: you **must** do Step 1 **before** Step 2

Step 1 ➡ Step 2

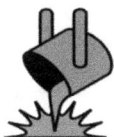

Tool #1

Talk

Grab one of your favorite friends

In-person

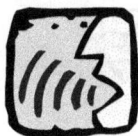

Text

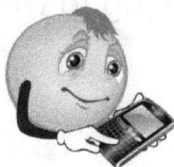

Phone

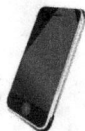

Either way..... You're *talking!*

IMPORTANT:

Talk about your *feelings*, **not** the situation!

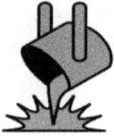

Tool #2

Do A Dump & Destroy

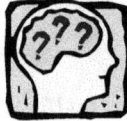

This is one of my secret weapons!

Here's what you need:

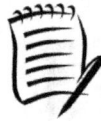

- ✓ A piece of paper
- ✓ Something to write with

1) Start writing

2) *DO NOT* READ IT

3) *Destroy IT!*

It WON'T work with a computer

It requires you to use paper!

This is different from "Journaling"....

with Dumping –

The goal = Just get it out!

Reading IT = *reloads it!*

It also works *really well* when**...

1)   You can't **fall asleep**
because your *mind racing*

2)   You **wake up** at night &
your mind is racing!

**IMPORTANT:

You must go write in ***another*** room for it to work.

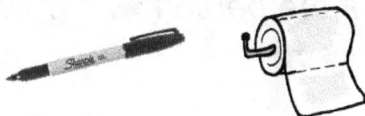

TIP: Use a sharpie & toilet paper, flush
when done. No one will ever read that!

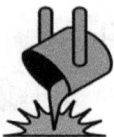

Tool #3

Empty Chair Method

When you don't have anyone

or you can't get a hold of someone

Use this tool!

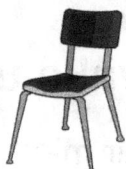

You start talking to the

"Empty Chair"

As if the person was there!

It is a great way to VENT without

getting in trouble for what you say!

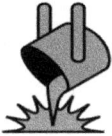 **Tool #4**

Get ACTIVE!

There are many ways to do this!

Walk

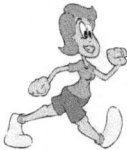

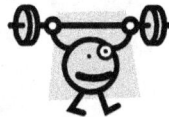

Any Kind of Exercise

Climb the Stairs

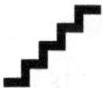

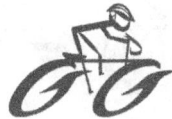

Bike

Push Ups

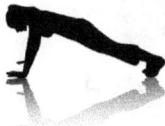

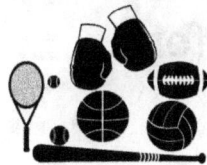

Sports

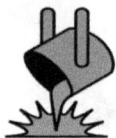

Tool #5

Music

For this tool to work, you MUST:

you **DO more** than just listen!

Dance = Any time you are *moving* to music!

ging = Doesn't mean you *can*
or
KNOW the words!

Perform = Play a real **instrument**
or
AIR guitar / drums

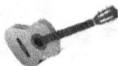

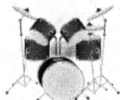

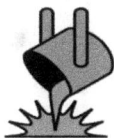

Tool #6

Punch n Dump!

There are **2** ways to do this:

1) Use a real punching bag.

Don't have one?

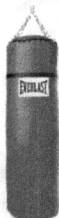

You can make one using a pillow!

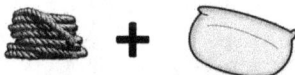

2) Air Boxing!

You must ***be sure*** to do this in a

place where it is SAFE.

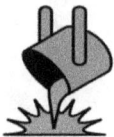 **Tool #7**

Let It Out!

When stress builds up…

Sometimes a good cry or a good laugh

is needed to *let it out!*

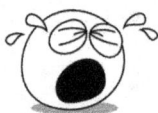**Cry**

It's perfectly okay to

let the tears flow.

(Even for guys)

Laugh

Watch a funny show

Try Laughter Yoga

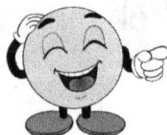

80

Here's a few more tools –

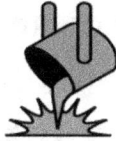

- Tear up an old phone book or a bunch of paper

- Wash the car

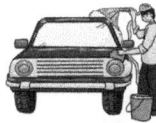

- Do some coloring!

- Clean the house!

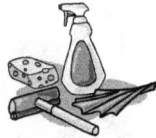

- Do some jumping jacks!

- Scream in a car or another safe place

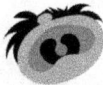

- Constructive Destruction – break something on PURPOSE!

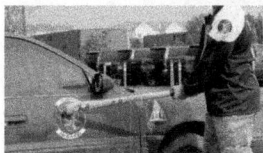

Can you think of other ways for you to:

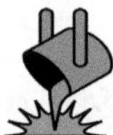

RELEASE what's there!

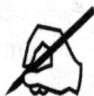

(Use another piece of paper if you need more room!)

Remember -

This step is one that is active...

(DOES require activity or muscles!)

Selfness

A New Approach to Self-Care!

What Is SELFNESS?

Many years ago,

I was running a therapy group

with patients at the hospital.

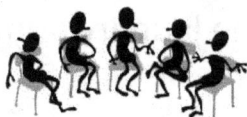

It was here that **SELFNESS** was born!

I had a patient I'll call Sue (not real name!)

who was a single mom -

struggling & *feeling overwhelmed.*

I asked her to identify **1** thing

she could **do** for herself tonight.

Her response:

"I couldn't do anything for me."

"I have to get the kids fed,

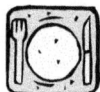

get them bathed & to bed,

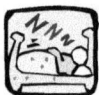

& the laundry done."

I gently nudged her to think of something

to 'do for herself' that would

FIT *around those things.*

Her response:

"I couldn't –

I've got too much to do."

I'd spent several years working

in a women's trauma program.

One of the **self-care**

foundations we used:

The Oxygen Mask!

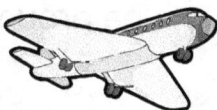

Since most had never flown, I explained:

"When the oxygen masks drop

from the ceiling & you have a

child or adult who needs help –

Put the MASK ON YOURSELF first,

then help them."

Sue immediately stated:

"Oh, I could never do that."

"I would put it on my children first."

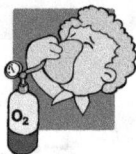

To which I responded-

"*Then* you won't be around for the kids,

because you'd pass out

before you get yours on

& *they can't help you.*"

Sue stuck to her answer:

"*I'd still do them* **1st**

What? Did I hear her **right?**

Her response did not make

sense to me so I asked why she

wouldn't **put it on herself first.**

She said:

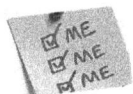

"That would be selfish."

I remember thinking

'Quick Carol,

you've got to **HELP** her get this.'

Thank goodness my Higher Power helped
&
I quickly came up with my own reply:

"NO-

that'd be practicing SELFNESS

which is very different from selfish."

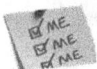

"*Selfish* is when we want **other people**

to **DO** *what we want.*

SELFNESS is when

we *take care of ourselves* **1st**

so we can be there to

take care of others

who may be needing us!"

When I asked the group if

this made sense…

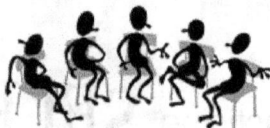

To my surprise,

they all said yes, **even Sue!**

So I checked with her one last time….

"Sue, *who'd* you put the mask on *first*?"

She answered with a loud:

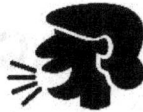

"MYSELF!"

SELFNESS was born that day!

It doesn't get any **simpler than that!**

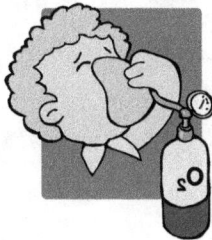

We MUST take care of ourselves

1st

IF we want to be around

to take care of others!!!!

Join me in *making a commitment* to

PRACTICE SELFNESS
EVERYDAY!

Improving

Communication

The Basics!

I'd like to start by reviewing some basics

which I've taken from my book-

"Transforming Illness to Wellness"

If I could teach only **1** skill to people

this is it!

I believe the **QUALITY** of our life

is greatly influenced

by the **QUALITY** of our

communication skills.

It is impossible to be effective

without communication skills!

There are **3** basic styles
of communication:

Aggressive

Assertive

Passive

Aggressive: My needs & wants are all
that matters! It's *MY* way.

Passive: My needs & wants aren't that
important. I *WON'T* say anything

Assertive: My needs & wants are just as
important as your needs &
wants are. *I'll let you know!*

WAIT!

I forgot the 4th one!!

Passive-aggressive

I use to be the queen of this!

This is the **MOST** *DAMAGING*
to our relationships

Because it leaves a feeling they're
NOT BEING honest with us.

With this approach
Behaviors speak louder than words!

Examples:

#1 - Rather than *tell the waitress*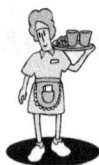

the service was poor

I don't leave a tip!

#2 - When you ask, "What's wrong?"

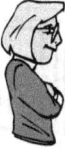

I say **"*nothing*"**

Yet, you can tell by my

tone & body language

"*something*" is!

#3 - Instead of me *telling you I'm angry*:

I **slam** doors & drawers,

make a lot of noise,

purposely do things to annoy you!

#4 - I communicate by ***what I don't say***!

the **silent treatment** showing up late,

or **_not calling_** when I'm supposed to!

It's like someone trying to SNEAK IN
to your home
through the **BACK**

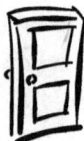

rather than walk in thru the front

Another way I like to have people
"see" communication:

Imagine we are both *sitting at the table.*

We are sitting across from one another.

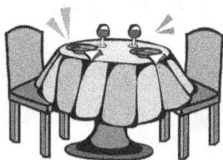

How would *you prefer* to
be 'served'?

- I **shove** everything at you!
    (aggressive)

- I **set it** on the table in front of you
    so you can take what you want.
    (assertive)

- I **don't put anything** on the
    table, leaving you with nothing.
    (passive)

    or

- I set it in front of you then **take it**,

    pretending it was never there to start!
    (passive-aggressive)

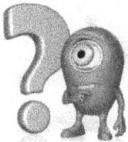

Which one best describes YOU?!

Communication is the single most
    important tool for **LIFE!**

Next:

6 Steps to Better Communication!

Talking Made Simple!

Regardless of what approach you're using,

being a **Caregiver** requires we be

Assertive

Anything other than this
will NOT WORK.....

It is critical you start to

PRACTICE these **6 simple steps**:

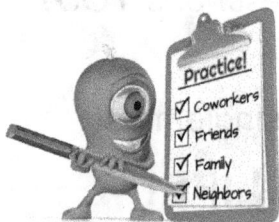

with co-workers

with friends

with neighbors & family

Practice them *away* from being a

Caregiver!

You don't wait until you're on **Titanic**

to *practice your new swimming skills!*

Purposely

Repeat

Activities

Critical

To

Improving

Core

Elements

© 2019 & licensed by Well YOUniversity, LLC
Taken from "WordTools"

Step #1

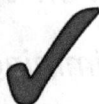 **Timing**

Ever had someone try to talk with you

WHEN your mind was *somewhere else?*

Don't make the same mistake…..

ASK first:

> *"Do you have a moment to talk?"*
>
> *or*
>
> *"Is this a good time to talk?"*

Respect their answer

If they say **NO** – you can ask:

> *"When would be a better time for you?"*
>
> *or*
>
> *"Okay, I'll check with you later."*

Don't push it! *No* means try again later.

Step #2

YOU ⟶ **I**

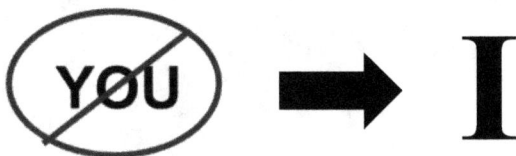

"**YOU**" is like an invisible **pointing** finger….

It's an attacking word!

Start all conversations with "**I**"

TRY: *I'm* angry.

or

I feel like *I'm* not being listened to.

STAY AWAY from:

"**You** made me mad"

or

"**You** don't listen to me."

When people feel **less defensive,**

they **hear more** of what you say!

Step #3

????

Ask a question, *rather than* **accuse**

TRY:

"What happened? I was getting worried."

or

"Is everything okay? I started to get concerned."

or

"Why didn't I hear from you?"

STAY AWAY from:

"You're late."

or

"You didn't show up on time."

or

"You didn't call me."

When people feel **accused** —

they *SHUT DOWN!*

Step #4

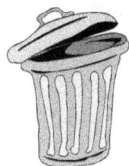

Always...Never...Everybody

They are fighting words!

When we use them, we **instantly** put people

on the defensive.

I call these **'trash can'** words.

Leave them in the trash can!!!

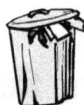

TRY:

> *"**It seems** like we always go there."*
>
> *or*
>
> ***It seems** to never get done.*

STAY AWAY from:

> *"We always go there."*
>
> *or*
>
> *"It never gets done."*

105

Step #5

What Do You See?

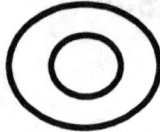

Tire	**Lifesaver**
Doughnut	**Inner Tube**
Cheerio	**Bagel**

Sure, we could *argue* about it.

The truth is we would BOTH be right!

2 people can look at the **SAME thing**

& *see it* differently.

We may not agree with them,

however, we must respect their position.

As I like to say: *Agree to disagree!*

Step #6

The
Great
Escape!

Finish off your sentence with

"……right now."

People are willing to **let you go now**

thinking there will be **a 'later'!**

TRY:

*"I'm not able to talk about it **right now.**"*

*"I'm not interested **right now**"*

STAY AWAY from:

" I don't want to talk about it."

"I'm not interested."

What *NOT* To Say

The **6 Steps** you just learned will apply across ALL areas of your life!

These are *universal tools!*

What *NOT* to say.

They are the following:

> You need to…
>
> Why don't you…
>
> Isn't it time you…
>
> How could you…
>
> What's wrong with you?
>
> You should….
>
> Didn't you know…
>
> I don't want to…
>
> What's your problem?
>
> "I told you…

What TO SAY

Here are some things to *say instead:*

Help me understand …

How are you doing?

Is there a reason…

Have you thought about….

How's that working for you?

I was wondering….

I was thinking about you ….

I'm confused…

I am not able to…

"I don't know if you are aware of this…"

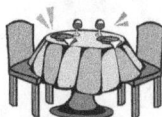

What to say = *putting stuff on the table!*

What* NOT *to say = shoving stuff
across the table at me!

Wrap Up!

Congratulations!

You now have the "tools" to

become a

Stress Master!

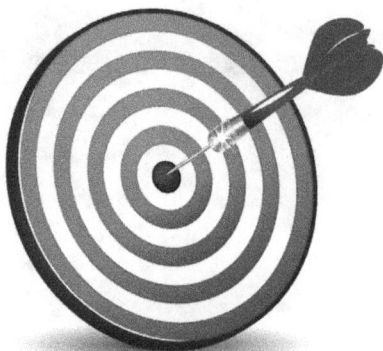

More importantly,

You can now MANAGE

your **work** **stress!**

It doesn't have to **RUIN**

the career you love.

You don't always get to be in

control

of your day...

Sometimes,

You just have to play the cards you get.

YOU

are **100% responsible** for *your response*

Part 1: Now You See It!

So,

There are **2** ways I got you to

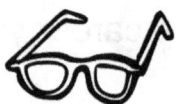

STRESS

Way # 1

Things happen in life that
shake a person up

And…

Just like the pressure
BUILT UP
in the bottle…

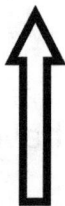

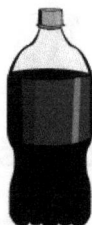

STRESS builds up *inside people!*

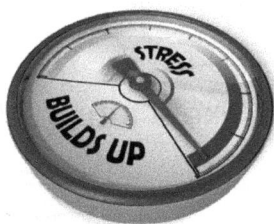

And once the *STRESS gets built up*

It stays there...

It won't go away on its own.

The **STRESS** doesn't go anywhere

UNTIL

we *do something to*

Let

It

Out!

Way #2

People are just like a tub:

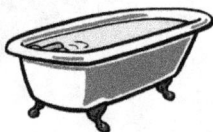

1) Your **STRESS** level starts to rise

& it will keep rising until it is…

shut off!

2) *YOU* only have *so much room -*

YOU can only hold so much

STRESS

until *YOU* will be at

OVERFLOW!!!

And how it won't go away

until we…

release it!

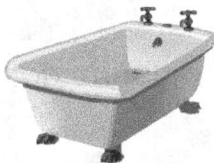

Part 2: Now You Don't!

There are **2** steps to the

DO*60* System™

Step 1 -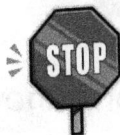

the level from **RISING!**

Step 2 -

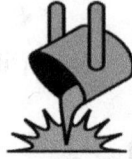

RELEASE so the level drops!

➤ **Each step** must be done *in order...*

Step 1 ➡ Step 2

➤ **Each step** must be done *60 Secs.*

Remember:

Most everyone in the world

gets it **wrong!**

They don't know to **DO** Step 2

Now **you** know the secret!

Bonus Tool

I created this tool for my patients &

discovered I **needed** it more!

If you start **feeling overwhelmed,**

I want you to use this:

The Serenity Prayer Stress Tool!

#1 Make a list of ALL the things that are stressing you out.

#2 Using the worksheet on the next page, place the things from your list in the appropriate section.

#1 Fold the paper on the line and **RIP IT IN HALF**. Get rid of what you CAN'T do anything about!

I have also created a couple

mini posters!

This way you can rip / cut them ✂
out of the book

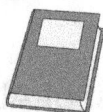

And put them up on your fridge, computer,
or wherever you'll see them!

This will help reinforce the
new tools you're trying to
get good at using!

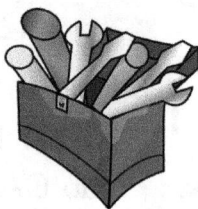

The Serenity Prayer Stress Tool!

Grant me the **serenity** to accept the things
I cannot change:

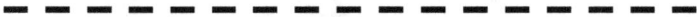

_____

_____

_____

_____

– – – – – – – – – – – – – – – – – – –

The **courage** to change the things I can:

_____

_____

_____

_____

And the **wisdom** to know the difference!

Intentionally blank

DO*60* System™-

Step 1 -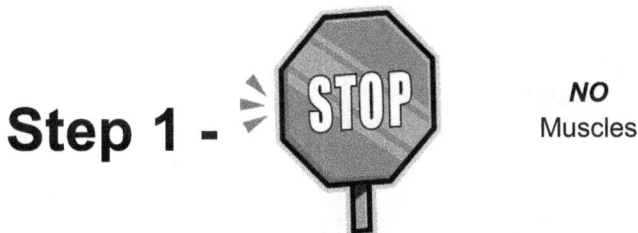

NO Muscles

the level from **RISING!**

Step 2 -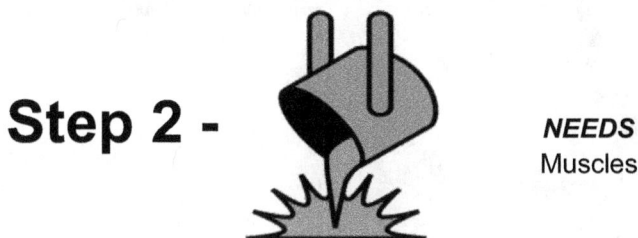

NEEDS Muscles

RELEASE so the level drops!

➢ **Each step** must be done *in order...*

Step 1 ➡ Step 2

➢ **Each step** must be done *60 Secs...*

Intentionally blank

124

The 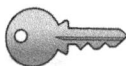 's to success!

#1 Try out each one.

(**even if** you don't think

it will work for you!)

#2 Do 60 Seconds.

(if you can go longer – **do it!**

30 secs. **is better than** none!

#3 Keep a list.

(write down tools that end

up working **best for you**)

#4 Have more than 1!

(don't set yourself up to fail

the **more tools** the better!)

Intentionally blank

The Stressometer

I find when I try to go to sleep, my mind just keeps racing about things.

1	2	3	4	5	6	7
Not at all						All the time

I find my appetite changes, I'm either eating more or eating less.

1	2	3	4	5	6	7
Not at all						All the time

I find myself getting really angry over the littlest things.

1	2	3	4	5	6	7
Not at all						All the time

I find I am having increased health issues. (ie. migraines, pain, & digestive)

1	2	3	4	5	6	7
Not at all						All the time

I find my relationship is being impacted by what goes on at work / home.

1	2	3	4	5	6	7
Not at all						All the time

Total: _____

**Use key – page 14

127

Intentionally blank

Want to Speed Up Your Progress?

StressMastery
Learn To Take Control Of Stress

Join Carol for this

FREE

Fast Start Training!

(Sells For $297.00)

You know the **DO60™ System** –

Now it's time to learn the 5 keys to

being an unstoppable Stress Master!

Sign Up Now!

StressYOUniversity.com/Caregivers

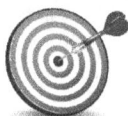

Sign Up For

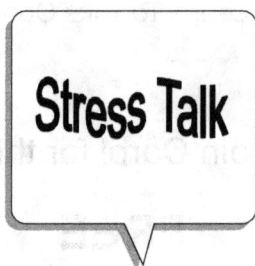

This 5 minute video newsletter will give you

more tips, tools, & rules for taking control of…

STRESS!

Sign up at:

StressYOUniversity.com/Stress-Talk

Carol's Other Resources

A Nationally Syndicated Wellness Series:

The WELL YOU Show

Mondays @ 6pm, Sundays @ 8am

Watch at: www.PrincetonTV.org

Catch past episodes at

www.TheWellYouShow.com

Want More Tools?!

Carol has written more "tool" books!

If you need help:

- ✓ Losing weight
- ✓ Dealing with anger
- ✓ Managing health issues

Take a look at the next few pages…

TRANSFORMING ILLNESS TO WELLNESS

Two Weeks to Transform Your Life!

CAROL L. RICKARD, LCSW

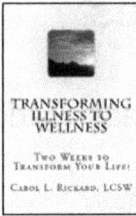

Chronic illness doesn't exclude you from having wellness. Get a blueprint to follow for taking back control of your health!

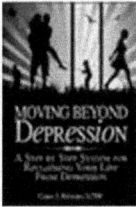

MOVING BEYOND DEPRESSION

A Step by Step System for Reclaiming Your Life From Depression

Carol L. Rickard, LCSW

Are you sick & tired of feeling sick & tired? This is a step by step system for reclaiming your life from depression.

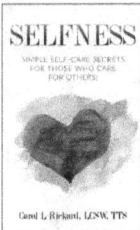

SELFNESS

SIMPLE SELF-CARE SECRETS FOR THOSE WHO CARE FOR OTHERS

Carol L. Rickard, LCSW, TTS

Self-care is often forgotten in this busy world. Carol offers simple and practical strategies to fit in to your busy life!

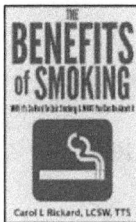

THE BENEFITS of SMOKING

Carol L. Rickard, LCSW, TTS

No – this is not promoting smoking! Instead, it provides the knowledge & the 'tools' to finally "Kick Cigarettes Butts"!

Available: amazon.com/author/carolrickard

ANGER

A Simple & Practical Approach for Those Who Need A Better Way of Dealing With It!

Carol I Rickard, LCSW, TTS

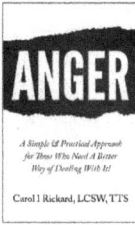

ANGER - one of the most powerful emotions there is. Learn how to manage it instead of it managing you!

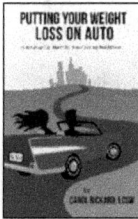

PUTTING YOUR WEIGHT LOSS ON AUTO

by CAROL RICKARD LCSW

Losing weight doesn't have to be complicated! Learn the *7 Laws of Lasting Weight Loss* a car can teach us. Guaranteed to work!

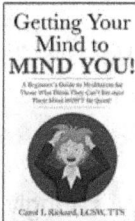

Getting Your Mind to **MIND YOU!**

Carol I. Rickard, LCSW, TTS

Your mind *is not* supposed to be quiet! Learn how mediation really works & change your life forever!

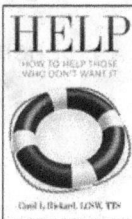

HELP

HOW TO HELP THOSE WHO DON'T WANT IT

Carol I. Rickard, LCSW, TTS

Do you find yourself struggling with what to say or how to help someone you care about? Learn how to say it & what to do!

Available: amazon.com/author/carolrickard

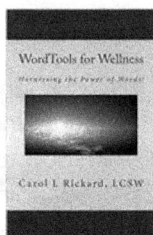

WordTools for Wellness
Harnessing the Power of Words!

Carol J. Rickard, LCSW

WordTools

What are words tools?
They are acronyms with purpose & meaning!

They are officially called *Artinyms™*, which is Sanskrit for "describe".

On the back of each wordtool is a question for you to answer should you choose to!

We have **4 different versions:**

Wellness Vol. 1 & 2,   *Self-Esteem* Vol. 1 & 2
Business Vol. 1 & 2,   *Athletes* Vol. 1

Examples:

The
Only
Day
Afforded
You!

A
Deliberate
Adjustment
Providing
Transformation

Daringly
Recognize
Experiences
As
Mine

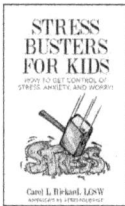

NEW RELEASE!!!!
Kid these days have to deal with so much stress. This makes sure they have the tools to succeed!!

We have three different versions of adult stress books because life circumstances can be different for each..

Choose the one that *best fits* your situation!

Caregiver

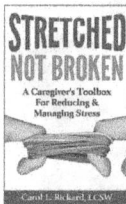

Research has shown caregivers are the MOST vulnerable. Learn quick, simple, practical tools for reducing and managing it.

Stress Eater

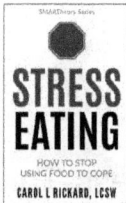

Do you find yourself eating when under stress? Get the tools & knowledge needed to break away from any old habits.

General

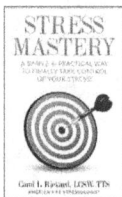

STRESS... It's all around us and NOT getting any less! Get the system Carol has taught to 1,000's & finally take control!

To Contact Carol:

Please feel free to reach out if you have questions or comments!

Email:

Carol@StressYOUniversity.com

Phone:

888 LifeTools

(543-3866)

Sign Up for Stress Talk:

StressYOUniversity.com/Stress-Talk

www.ingramcontent.com/pod-product-compliance
Lightning Source LLC
Chambersburg PA
CBHW060905280326
41934CB00007B/1188